A Mouthful of TRUTH

{ the real deal on food and eating }

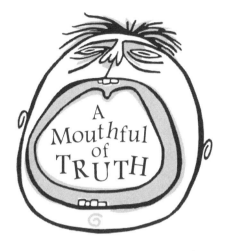

A
Mouthful
of
TRUTH

{ the real deal on food and eating }

Albert Eiler and Julie Long

A Not Long Book

Book design and illustrations by Patricia Tsagaris.
www.pinkhausdesign.com

ISBN 978-0-9843185-1-3

{ We are all dietetic sinners; only a small percent of what we eat
nourishes us; the balance goes to waste and loss of energy. }

~William Osler

Contents

Can you handle the truth?

This book will challenge your character. It may even provide a rude awakening. It is written with a level of directness that is missing in the health industry, where all too often either the message or its delivery is softened for the sake of marketability (and in doing so the truth gets compromised). I have more faith in you than that. I think you want the truth. I think you can handle the truth.

One day not too long ago, I spoke to a local community group about putting together a Group Challenge Program to improve daily living performance, promote general health and create leaner bodies. In response to a remark I made about overweight and obese bodies, a clearly overweight woman said, "Our bodies are just a shell God made for us while we're on earth." Many others in the group chimed in their agreement. "That may be," I said, "but my guess is that God did not intend for us to abuse our 'shells' with gluttony and disrespect."

To play down the importance of the physical body is just one of many ways we excuse the fact that so many of us have lost self-control. This loss of self-control to the point of not being able to control our food intake saddens me. And it happens at all socioeconomic levels. Mr. Lead can run a very successful business, have a big house and a vacation home, yet struggle with his very own self-control. His employees, from the top executives to the janitor, struggle with this same lack of control. And everyone's poor eating behaviors are causing our healthcare costs to skyrocket from diseases that could be avoided.

For much of the history of the human race, obtaining food was a major struggle. Finding it and preparing it took time and effort. It still does in many cultures around the world. But for most Americans today, food is everywhere. And we reach for it without thought. We are overfed and yet undernourished. We eat for enjoyment and comfort, no longer for sustenance. Our lives are excessively busy, and prepackaged, engineered, processed foods are so much faster. The funny thing is, so much of that time we're saving is used up trying to cover up our inadequacies with material diversions. We search out clothing to make us appear trimmer than we are or depend on prescriptions to mask the underlying problem, instead of simply focusing on the things that would actually make us leaner and healthier.

There's something else at work, as well. A sense of entitlement. Along with all sorts of material things we feel we deserve, we now demand food that is convenient, fast, cheap, fills us to capacity, and tastes up to ridiculous flavor standards (everything must be salty, savory or sweet). But there's a price to pay to be able to eat this way. That price is our health and the cost of trying to fix it. It turns out we can't have it all. Imagine that.

We've eaten ourselves into quite a state. But the good news is that in most cases we can eat ourselves right back out of it, back into good health. What's more, the method is simple. It's not rocket science. It's not even food science. It's simple common sense. Many of you already know what to do, you simply choose not to do it. This book, I hope, will change your mind.

I understand that it's difficult to change a culture, and painful – emotionally and physically – to be in the midst of a struggle. But rather than place blame on external factors (too busy, too poor, etc.) or internal factors (bad genes, hormones, etc.), accept that you are responsible for your state of health.

Some people won't like hearing what this book has to say. You can dislike the message and its delivery, but you cannot dismiss its validity. You can try to avoid the truth, saying it's too "drastic," or not "realistic" because it doesn't fit into your "lifestyle." But here's the biggest truth you must accept:

Nutrition isn't a variable — it is the constant in the equation for health. Thus you must be willing to adjust your lifestyle to accommodate nutrition.

Refrain from dismissing this and other truths presented in this book until you try them and realize their effectiveness. If you live with them and live by them, you will live well. Some of what you are asked to accept and do will feel difficult at first. But rather than find a reason why it can't be done, I ask you to simply accept that it must be done.

— Albert Eiler

{ Life expectancy would grow by leaps and bounds
if green vegetables smelled as good as bacon. }
~Doug Larson

Truth #1:
You didn't get this way eating broccoli.

"I eat healthy foods. Why can't I lose weight?"

As a nation we pay more attention to health than ever before. And yet, we're unhealthier than at any point in modern history. Children born in the year 2000 will be the first generation to live shorter lives than the generation before. So what's going on?

Here's the simple truth: You think you eat nutritiously, but you don't. You make smart choices some of the time. Maybe even most of the time. But not enough of the time.

There is a nutrimental threshold you must cross in order to see positive results. And to fall short of that minimum and still expect success is like being dropped in ten feet of water and hoping to survive by swimming up only nine feet. It's not going to work. You've got to swim all the way up. You've got to break the surface. Then from there you can decide if you want to keep just your nose above water or try to walk on water. But first, you have to not drown.

In today's America, we've become accustomed to being rewarded for any minimal effort. Everyone gets a trophy! But nutrition doesn't conform to that norm. A slight improvement in your eating habits might bring minimal improvements in health, such as small reductions in cholesterol or blood pressure. But it's unlikely that you'll experience vast health improvements, nor will you see ample weight loss or a lean body, until you make significant modifications in your eating habits.

It's not enough to think about it. It's not enough to try. You must do.

{ True wisdom consists in not departing from nature and in molding our conduct according to her laws and model. }

~Seneca

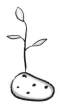

Truth #2:
The potato isn't the problem.

No one gets fat from eating a potato. It doesn't matter that it's a starchy carbohydrate. The potato has been part of various diets throughout civilization without anyone getting fat. Until recently. But the potato isn't the problem.

The problem is how you prepare the potato. You take a natural, unprocessed whole food and then you sabotage it with butter, sour cream and bacon bits. Or you let someone else sabotage it by deep frying it in oil (sometimes first breading it), and then you sabotage it some more by drenching it in sugary ketchup or processed cheese sauce.

You do the same thing with lettuce. You assault a simple salad with loads of bottled dressing, croutons and cheese topping and then pat yourself on the back for having eaten some greens. Meanwhile, the calories can very easily soar from 300 to 900 with very little added nutritional value.

This is the Western diet: small amounts of produce and whole grains overshadowed by highly processed foods, refined grains, and added fat, salt and sugar. And it's making us sick. The Western diet has been linked to diseases like obesity, type 2 diabetes, cardiovascular disease and cancer. Other cultures don't have these diseases, even in cases where their diets are high in natural fat or centered around complex carbohydrates (like the potato). Western diseases don't exist for these cultures. Until, that is, they start eating the Western diet.

When we ruin our food, we ruin our bodies.

{ As for butter versus margarine, I trust cows more than chemists. }
~Joan Gussow

Truth #3:
If you can't fish it, grow it or butcher it, don't eat it.

You don't have to start your own farm, or start hunting and fishing. But almost everything you eat should be found either in the ground or grazing on it, or in the woods or the water. This is the test. This is how you'll know you are eating whole foods and not derivatives or extractions or concoctions manufactured by food scientists.

You won't find ethoxylated diglycerides on a farm. These and other ingredients are added during processing. The more a food is processed, the more it tends to lose nutrients and in some cases gain toxic chemicals. In addition, processed food becomes more easily absorbed into our bodies, which can cause problems with our insulin and fat metabolism. Processed foods are at the root of our nation's food issues as a whole. It's best to simply avoid them.

When shopping for groceries, you'll have the best luck in avoiding processed foods if you shop on the perimeter of the store. While some processed items do lurk here – bakery goods, lunchmeats, sugary yogurts – in general, the perimeter is home to many whole foods (produce, meat and seafood) because they are perishable and it's more convenient for the grocer to regularly restock them. A Twinkie can sit on a shelf in the middle of the store for ages and not go bad. You can't fish, grow or butcher a Twinkie.

In the center aisles of the grocery store, focus your shopping on whole grains, oats, legumes, lentils, etc. And if you can't always follow the "farm it or forget it" rule, at least choose foods with only a few ingredients instead of a paragraph-long list. The shorter the list, the closer that food is to its original whole-food state and the less it's been processed into something you'd never be able to fish, grow or butcher.

Know what's in processed food:

- *88% of juices exceed the recommended sugar threshold, and 23% contain high fructose corn syrup.*
- *More than 75% of white bread products contain high fructose corn syrup.*
- *44% of milk products contain added sugar.*
- *14% of yogurts exceed the recommended sugar threshold, 26% contain high fructose corn syrup, and one-quarter contain artificial colors that are under review to be banned.*
- *13% of baby juices contain ingredients that are not allowed in food in the European Union.*
- *28% of crackers and 11% of cold cereals contain hydrogenated oils or trans fat.*
- *75% of fruit snacks contain added colors.*

Source: Good Guide processed food database www.GoodGuide.com

Truth #4:
Savory, salty and sweet are scarce in nature.
(So make them scarce in your diet.)

Fat, salt and sugar are not overly abundant in the wild. But outside of nature, you'll find them everywhere. And with good reason. Food manufacturers rely on the triple-combination to make processed foods highly palatable. If you put enough fat, salt and sugar on it, even a piece of cardboard will taste good.

You know that high amounts of these ingredients are not good for us. They make us fat and they make us sick. But what you also need to realize is that fat, salt and sugar alter the brain's chemistry in ways that compel us to overeat. They stimulate dopamine and opioids so that the brain craves more. So even when you're full, you're not satisfied. It's a proven neurological response that the food industry leverages to get you to eat more. Don't fall for it.

Do yourself a favor and make savory, salty and sweet

foods scarce in your diet. Enjoy these flavors when they occur naturally, such as the fat in nuts and the sugar in fruits.

{ Did you ever stop to taste a carrot? Not just eat it, but taste it? You can't taste the beauty and energy of the earth in a Twinkie. }
~Astrid Alauda

Truth #5:
The formula for healthy eating is simple.

Healthy Meal =
protein + vegetable + starch/grain + fat + dessert (fruit!)

Follow the simple equation above and you can cre-ate a nutritious meal with a multitude of food options. Pick a protein such as chicken, fish, meat, eggs or even tofu (a minimally processed alternative to animal protein). Pair the protein with vegetables – anything from salad greens to a medley of peppers. Add a side of starch or grains. This might be a sweet potato, brown rice, chickpeas or lentils. Accent with a bit of natural fat, such as olive oil, nuts or seeds. And for your sweet tooth, end the meal with a piece of fruit.

If you wanted, you could save some of the nuts or fruit and eat them as a snack. If snacking leads you down a bumpy road of processed sweets and junk food, then the simple solution is don't snack. There's nothing wrong with only eating three square meals a day. Yes, there are metabolic advantages to eating five or six small meals per day. But this idea of frequent snacking has opened up a world of abuse. Instead of naturally nourishing options, people are choosing unfavorable foods and completely overriding any metabolic benefit from frequency eating. The state of health would not be threatened if everyone converted to consuming three nutrient-rich, non-processed meals per day.

As for portion sizes, here are some good rules of thumb: A portion of protein, starch/grain or fruit should fit in the palm of your hand. A portion of vegetables should be the size of your hand (or more). And when it comes to fats, think drizzle or sprinkle versus drench or load.

You should know that the whole idea of portion control was invented to restrain our intake of unhealthy foods. If you are eating wholesome foods prepared nutritiously – baked, steamed or grilled with a bit of olive oil and spices – you really don't have to worry about your portion sizes. You would be hard pressed to over eat on broccoli, lentils or grilled cod.

If you'd like to see examples of meals that pack a powerful wholesome punch with all natural foods, we've included some menus in the appendix of this book.

Truth #6:
Food is fuel.

You must start eating for fuel, not for fun. We're not saying you can't enjoy your food. But you've got to start valuing food for how it makes you feel physically instead of emotionally. Taking comfort in crap and joy from junk is not the way to go. The comfort and joy derived from food are all too short-lived, and then you're left with a body that feels (and looks) lousy.

There are so many other things in life from which to take comfort and joy. Become a participant in life rather than a spectator eating nachos in the stands. When you start exploring other outlets, you'll take the focus off food to fill the void.

Here's another interesting result of eating for fuel: As your body begins to feel better from the higher-quality food you are giving it, you actually start craving the healthy stuff. That's right, there will come a time (if you haven't experienced it already) when you'll actually prefer the taste of fresh whole foods. This is especially true if your vegetables and fruits come fresh from local farms.

Keep your fuel flavorful:

Have you bitten into a beautiful strawberry or tomato only to find it had no taste? Produce that is shipped thousands of miles is often specifically grown and harvested to withstand that transport. In doing so, it loses flavor. You'll be amazed at the enhanced taste (not to mention shelf life) when produce is freshly picked from local sources.

Shop at a farmers' market, buy a share of a CSA (community supported agriculture) farm, or even grow your own veggies — gardening is a great way to participate in life!

Truth #7:
Fast food is no excuse for *fat* food.

There's been a big spotlight on fast food merchandisers and the health horrors of our supersized-and-high-fructose-corn-syrup society. But guess what? We're not going to tell you not to eat fast food. (Surprised?) We'd be happier if you didn't but we know you are going to. So go ahead. But don't make the trip through the drive thru an excuse to abandon good eating habits. Man up and apply the Fish It, Grow It or Butcher It truth to your order.

"Wait," you argue, "I can't find healthy food at a fast food joint." Oh yes you can. Salad. Grilled chicken. Baked potato. Even a plain burger. Steer clear of the cheese, special sauce and high-fat dressings — and of course no fries.

If you're whining that we just took all the fun out of fast food, refer back to Truth #6.

{ Tell me what you eat, I'll tell you who you are. }
~Anthelme Brillat-Savarin

Truth #8:
You've got to eat clean to be lean.

Right about now you may be thinking, "Instead of giving up all the food I love, I'll just exercise more." If your only goal is to lose some weight, this might work to an extent. But you could still be open to health risks (we all know slender people who've had heart attacks or diabetes). And you definitely won't become the lean body you're envisioning. Exercise alone won't give you six-pack abs.

When it comes to obtaining and maintaining a lean body, exercise matters, to be sure. But food matters more. If you've ever wondered why, despite grunting through hundreds of abdominal crunches, you still have those love handles and belly fat, this is why. Yes, you're building muscles and a strong core – but it'll remain covered in a layer of fat unless and until you eat nutritiously.

Picture a pie chart divided between exercise, eating

clean and rest. For overall health, the pie is divided evenly between these three factors. If you have a greater concern for performance – maybe you're a professional athlete – then more emphasis must be placed on exercise (conditioning). But if, like most people, you desire a lean body, you must put a greater emphasis on eating right. It's not enough to head to the gym. You've got to head to the grocery store or the farmers' market and eat mindfully.

{ Desire is irrelevant. I am a machine. }
~The Terminator

Truth #9:
Hunger isn't the same as desire.

It is humbling how fortunate we are in our country today, particularly compared to societies – both past and present – that have struggled on a daily basis to gather enough food to survive. Compared to them, we are spoiled. Food has become an entitlement rather than a blessing. We live a gluttonous lifestyle that disrespects our ancestors and those currently struggling for sustenance. (Is it really necessary to have a soda and pretzels on a one-hour flight?)

Why must your taste buds be happy all the time? Why must you eat what you desire instead of what your body requires? Many of you reading this book don't know what true hunger feels like. If you still feel hungry after eating a healthy meal, eat a second helping of vegetables. If you don't want more broccoli, you're not hungry. You may be desirous of something, but you sure as heck aren't hungry.

{ … angel food cake, doughnuts, white bread and gravy
cannot build an enduring nation. }
~Martin H. Fischer

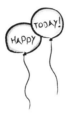

Truth #10:
Special occasions only occur occasionally.

Therefore, so must your special-occasion food choices. By definition that means infrequently. From time to time. Every once in a while.

Back in the days when most people prepared their own food, we might have occasionally made fried chicken or potato chips or cake. Now all these special occasion foods come readily available from nearby establishments, regardless of whether the occasion calls for them. So you must make the call. Does the occasion warrant this fattening, health-risk food?

If going out to dinner is not a special occasion – and for most of us it usually isn't – then you can't rationalize poor choices. Frankly, you're just not that special.

{ In general, mankind, since the improvement in cookery,
eats twice as much as nature requires. }
~Benjamin Franklin

Truth #11:
Full is a four letter word.
(So shut your mouth.)

You don't need to walk around famished. But satisfying your hunger is different than eating until you are full. Full means filled to capacity, unable to hold any more. This would apply if we were fueling ourselves for a long trek and the nourishment had to last us through a barren desert. But most of us don't have to worry where our next meal is coming from or when we can eat again. We'll eat again when we're hungry again. So once you've satisfied your hunger, stop eating. The ability to exercise restraint is a sign of personal fortitude.

Yes, what you're eating is tasty. But we live in a land of plenty. You can find more tasty stuff later. For now, just shut your mouth.

{ As a child my family's menu consisted of two choices:
take it or leave it. }
~Buddy Hackett

Truth #12:
It doesn't cost more to eat healthy.
(So there goes that excuse.)

There's a lot of talk that it's cheaper to order off the value menu than it is to make a meal at home. There is a notion circulating that some people aren't eating healthy foods simply because they can't afford them. That's bull. You're not eating processed food for economical reasons. You're eating it because you think it's tasty and it's more convenient than making a meal from scratch. You may tell yourself it's just too expensive to eat nutritiously, but that's really just an excuse to eat poorly.

In actuality, many healthy foods are not more expensive than processed foods. Take a trip to the grocery store and buy the following whole foods: oats, eggs, natural peanut butter and fresh strawberries (for breakfast), and ground beef, sweet potatoes, frozen green beans and almonds (for dinner). You can create two nourishing meals of approximately 500 calories each, and spend only $1.26 per person for breakfast and $1.88 per person for dinner. (You can find the cost analysis details in the appendix of this book.)

That's pretty darn affordable for a wholesome, well-balanced meal. Even if you were able to find fast-food meals with comparable cost and calorie totals, the nutrient density would pale by comparison.

Of course, you certainly can spend much more for healthy foods, choosing prime beef, sashimi-grade fish or exotic fruits. But the point is, eating wholesome foods while staying within budget can be done.

One last point about the cost of food: Americans spend less than 10% of our incomes on food. That's less than any other country. The richest nation in the world will gladly spend a sizable chunk of money on material goods but we don't place enough value on sustenance – on our health – to invest in quality food.

{ One of the very nicest things about life is the way we must regularly stop whatever it is we are doing and devote our attention to eating. }

~Luciano Pavarotti

Truth #13:
You have time to cook.

Are you one of those people who complain about not having time to cook, and then rush through your take-out dinner so you can sit on the couch watching TV? Yes, cooking takes time. You've got to make the grocery list, shop and then prepare the meal. So what? Get over it. You can make up the time somewhere else.

Do you realize that since the rise of the internet we've all somehow found the time to be on our computers on average two hours a day? If we can find time for social media, surfing and games, we can steal half an hour to prepare a meal. Slow down and make a conscious decision about your food. You'll find the benefits permeate into the rest of your life.

If you ever have the pleasure of driving through the rolling hills of Jamaica, you'll see some of the most beautiful bodies on earth: long, lean, vibrant. For many people there, the largest part of their day is spent harvesting and preparing their foods, instead of keeping up with the Joneses and accumulating material things. An entire movement, called Slow Food (www.slowfoodusa.org), formed around a similar recognition and works to counteract fast food and fast life. Don't knock it until you've tried it.

Slow down. Stop treating food with disregard. Take time to gather and prepare it with thoughtfulness, then bring your family together around the table (and turn off the cell phones). Relish the abundance nature provides and give thanks for the life forms sacrificed for our existence.

{ Reality must take precedence over public relations,
for Nature cannot be fooled. }
~Richard Feynman

Truth #14:
There is no super food to save you.

Instead of facing the truth about what you must do to eat nutritiously, many of you rationalize excuses for why you can't fit eating well into your lifestyle. Then you seek out some saving grace you can cling to in order to feel like you are doing something positive.

You drink the juice of an exotic super-berry but you snack on chips instead of an apple. You spend a fortune on Omega-3 fatty acids in a pill form, when you could just eat salmon and walnuts. You debate over the virtues of cage-free versus pastured, grass-fed versus locally raised, organic versus natural, and all the while you're sipping artificially sweetened soda.

Why do you have to make things so complicated? If only you could accept the simple truth. There is not one big move or quick fix you can take. There is only ongoing accountability and the daily choices you make. For food to play a prominent role in your health – which it must – you must apply the basic equation of eating naturally on a consistent basis.

{ To heal ourselves we must heal our planet, and to heal our planet we must heal ourselves. }
~Bobby McLeod

Truth #15:
It's not all about you.

The food choices you make day in and day out don't only affect your health. They impact the health of our food system and the environment. The more a food is processed, the more energy resources it wastes, not to mention wasteful packaging and production waste from the processing itself.

Much of the food we buy gets thrown away. If it is whole and natural it will decay and decompose. But when that food has been processed with chemical additives – like aspartame, MSG, fluoride, etc. – it leaches toxins into the underground watercourses, which can eventually spread neurotoxins into ponds, streams and lakes. The food chain then transfers these chemicals from one species to another. Insects also ingest and transfer the chemicals throughout our planet's biodiversity.

When you choose natural, unprocessed foods, you support healthy biology – in yourself and on our planet.

{ One's stomach is one's internal environment. }
~Samuel Butler

The truth shall set you free.

So there you have it. Fifteen food truths. Will you accept them and rethink your approach to eating? Will you take control of your actions and not allow food to dominate you? Will you break out of the prison of engineered, processed foods? Will you own the fact that we've become severely disrespectful of our bodies and our food chain?

Change is scary. There will be those who choose to ignore the truth and will continue to live a life of gluttony. But those people must understand that they cannot hide. It's all too clear that they lack self-control, dignity and respect for not only themselves but for others, for their actions will cost all of us more in the long run.

When you choose to accept the truths of this book, you may not immediately succeed in living by them. It takes time to modify a lifetime of habits and culture does not shift easily. But you will keep trying, because now you know the path that leads to significant change, the path to a lean, healthy being. And when you accept the truth, and begin living the truth, the truth shall set you free.

{ Food is power. Are you in control of yours? }

~John Jeavons

Sample Menus

Breakfast:	Lunch:	Dinner:
eggs	*chicken breast*	*cod*
green peppers	*broccoli*	*spinach leaves*
oatmeal	*chickpeas*	*lentils*
sunflower seeds	*peanuts*	*walnuts*
strawberries	*raspberries*	*kiwi*

Breakfast:	Lunch:	Dinner:
pork chop	*salmon*	*roast beef*
mushrooms	*salad greens*	*green beans*
quinoa	*brown rice*	*sweet potato*
flax seeds	*pistachio nuts*	*almonds*
blueberries	*blackberries*	*applesauce*

Portion Size Guidelines:

A portion of vegetables = hand-size or more
A portion of protein, starch/grain or fruit = palm-size
A portion of fat = a drizzle of oil or sprinkling of nuts/seeds

---

What about dairy?

Technically, it is processed, but compared to many foods, very minimally. Cow and goat products such as milk and yogurt are fantastic sources of naturally occurring calcium, as well as moderate sources of protein. (For those who experience lactose intolerance, there are many lactose-free products available.) Feel free to add a serving or two of dairy to your daily menu. But be sure to choose products that have no sugar added. And be cautious when it comes to cheese: While cottage cheese and ricotta can be suitable sources of protein, many other types of cheese are loaded with fat. High-fat cheeses should be used sparingly, similar to the way you would sprinkle your nuts or drizzle your oil.

Cost Analysis from Truth #12

Breakfast:

Oats: 42-oz container = $3
30 1/2-cup servings (150 cals per serving) = $.10/serving

Eggs: 1 dozen = $1.80
6 2-egg servings (160 cals per serving) = $.30/serving

Natural Peanut Butter: 16 oz jar = $3
28 1-Tbsp. servings (100 cals per serving) = $.11/serving

Fresh Strawberries: 1 lb container = $3
4 4-oz servings (44 cals per serving) = $.75/serving

TOTAL 454-CALORIE BREAKFAST = $1.26

Dinner:

Sweet Potatoes: 1 lb bag = $1.99
4 4-oz servings (150 cals per serving) = $.50/serving

Beef Ground Round: 1 lb = $3.99
4 4-oz servings (280 cals per serving) = $1/serving

Green Beans Frozen: 1 lb = $1
4 1-cup servings (45 cals per serving) = $.25/serving

Almonds: 16 oz jar = $4
32 1/2-oz servings (85 cals per serving) = $.13/serving

TOTAL 560-CALORIE DINNER = $1.88

Prices are from May 2010 from grocery stores in Pittsburgh, PA.

About the Authors

Albert Eiler is the president of Stick With It Fitness and ChangeRx, where he works closely with people at all levels of athletic ability, as well as special populations, either individually or though his Group Challenge Programs. Along with his team of experienced performance coaches, he has helped thousands of clients enhance their health and wellness through his *ChangeRx* methodology, which is centered on four principles: nutrition, conditioning, restoration and accountability. He instructs that no matter how deeply one delves into the topics of general health, human performance and body composition, the basic foundations of each core principle must be established and maintained. Contact him at aeiler@stickwithitfitness.com or visit www.changerxchallenge.com.

Julie Long is a freelance writer and published author. She credits her dietician mother for teaching her what a balanced meal looks like, and Albert Eiler for teaching her to be accountable for her own health. Her other books include *Fat, Dumb and Lazy,* a simple story for those who seek change, and *BABY: An Owner's Manual,* the operating instructions no baby should be delivered without. She is currently working on a novel entitled *The Growing Season*. Learn more about her on her blog and website: www.julielongwrites.com.

Made in the USA
Monee, IL
20 January 2021

58117025R00028